Glowing Skin Care

Unlock Flawless Skin and Youthful Vitality with Anti-Aging Power, Scar Revision, and Reinvented Skincare. Discover the Power of Potent Skin Elixirs.

By Kristin Hampton

Copyright © 2024 by Kristin Hampton

Disclaimer

The only objective of this book is to provide information; it is not meant to be used as a source of medical prescriptions or recommendations. It is important to note that the material included in this book is derived from the author's own experiences, research, and views. It is not intended to serve as a replacement for the advice, diagnosis, or treatment offered by a qualified medical professional. Before making any modifications to their skincare or wellness regimens, readers should discuss their options with a certified healthcare practitioner before making any changes.

This book's author and publisher do not make any claims or guarantees on the truth, applicability, suitability, or completeness of the information included within it. They expressly disclaim all guarantees, whether explicit or implied, as well as any claims about merchantability or suitability for any individual purpose. It is not possible to hold the author or publisher responsible for any loss or harm that may occur as a result of the utilization of the information that is included in this book.

While every effort has been taken to guarantee the accuracy of the material contained in this book, the author and publisher accept no responsibility for mistakes or omissions, or any consequences arising from the use of the information within.

About the Author

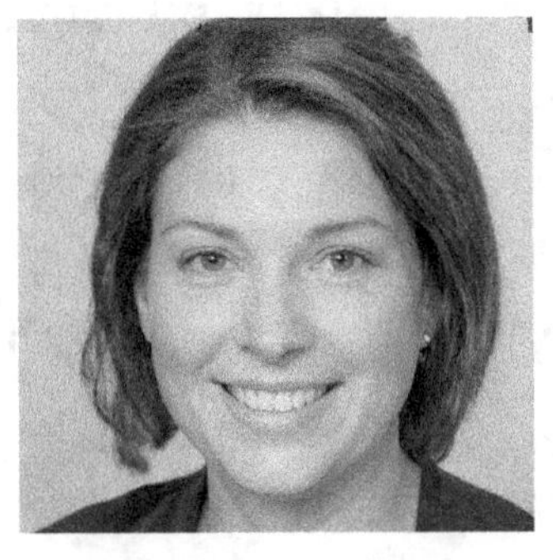 Kristin Hampton is a passionate advocate for healthy living and beauty, dedicated to empowering individuals to embrace their natural radiance. With a lifelong commitment to wellness and beauty practices, Kristin's journey has been guided by a deep passion for nurturing both the body and the soul.

Drawing upon her personal experiences and extensive research, Kristin shares her expertise in her book, "Glowing Skin Care." In this transformative guide, she explores the intersection of skincare and holistic well-being, offering readers practical insights and actionable advice to achieve radiant, glowing skin from the inside out.

Kristin's holistic approach to beauty extends beyond skincare products, encompassing nourishing lifestyle practices that promote vitality and longevity. From mindful nutrition and fitness to self-care rituals and stress management techniques, she believes in cultivating a holistic lifestyle that nurtures both inner and outer beauty.

In addition to her dedication to healthy living and beauty, Kristin finds joy and fulfilment in her role as a wife and partner. Together with her spouse, she navigates life's journey with love, laughter, and unwavering support.

Through her writing and advocacy, Kristin seeks to inspire others to embark on their own journey to radiant health and beauty. With her compassionate approach and genuine commitment to holistic well-being, she continues to make a positive impact, empowering individuals to embrace their natural beauty and live their best lives.

Table of Contents

Introduction

In the vast landscape of beauty and skincare, where trends come and go like fleeting seasons, the pursuit of radiant skin often feels like a maze, leaving us yearning for a guide that is not just effective but universally inclusive. Welcome to Glowing Skin Care, a transformative journey through the realms of skincare that transcends age, skin type, and ethnicity—a guide crafted for anyone seeking the secret to unlocking their skin's natural brilliance.

In these pages, you'll discover more than just a skincare routine; you'll find a companion for your odyssey toward luminosity. Whether you're a skincare novice seeking simplicity or a beauty enthusiast eager for new insights, this book is designed to meet you where you are. Imagine a roadmap that navigates you through the clutter, demystifying the world of beauty with relatable stories and empowering advice.

The essence of this book lies in its simplicity. No more overwhelming routines or complicated rituals; instead, you'll find straightforward, user-friendly guidance that adapts to your lifestyle. Together, we'll explore the fundamentals of skincare, embracing the belief that every individual, regardless of age, background, or skin type, deserves to revel in the glow of their skin.

This book is your invitation to a celebration of beauty in all its forms. Whether you're drawn to the simplicity of a daily routine, the joy of DIY masks, or the empowerment of embracing your unique skin tone, Glowing Skin Care has something for everyone.

So, if you're ready to embark on a journey towards radiant skin—one that is uncomplicated, inclusive, and tailored to your unique needs—turn the page and let the exploration begin.

Why Glowing Skin Matters

In the symphony of self-expression, our skin plays the lead, conducting a silent yet powerful narrative about who we are and how we feel. It's not just a canvas; it's a reflection of our inner vitality. Why Glowing Skin Matters, is more than a question—it's a statement about the transformative power of healthy, radiant skin and its profound impact on our self-confidence and overall well-being.

Imagine waking up every morning to a face that radiates not just external beauty but an inner vitality that lights up your entire being. It's not about conforming to societal standards but rather about embracing a version of yourself that exudes confidence, resilience, and self-love.

Glowing skin matters because it is a testament to a well-nurtured relationship with oneself. It's a journey where each skincare step becomes an act of self-care, a daily affirmation of self-worth. When your skin glows, it's as if your body whispers a secret to the world "I am here, I am vibrant, and I am taking care of myself."

Beyond aesthetics, the significance of glowing skin extends to the realms of mental and emotional well-being. Picture the confidence that comes with feeling comfortable in your skin, the assurance that radiates from within, and the positive energy that reverberates through every interaction. Glowing skin becomes a source of empowerment, fostering a sense of inner strength that transcends beauty norms.

Moreover, the pursuit of glowing skin is not about perfection but about embracing imperfections with grace. It's a journey that acknowledges the uniqueness of each individual, celebrating the diverse tapestry of skin tones and types. When we prioritize our skin's health, we are not merely indulging in a beauty ritual; we are investing in our overall wellness.

So, as we delve into the pages of Glowing Skin Care, remember that the quest for radiant skin is not a frivolous pursuit, it's a journey toward self-love, confidence, and well-being. So, let's explore the transformative power of glowing skin and discover how it can be a beacon of light on your path to a more radiant and empowered you.

How to Use This Book

Welcome to Glowing Skin Care! This book is your ultimate companion on the journey to achieving luminous, healthy skin and embracing your natural beauty. Here's your guide to navigating through each chapter and unlocking the secrets to radiant skin:

Know Your Skin: Start by getting to know your skin inside and out. Discover your skin type, learn about common concerns, and gain valuable insights into creating a personalised skincare routine that works for you.

Building Your Basics: Dive into the foundational elements of skincare, from cleansing and toning to protection. Master the essentials and lay the groundwork for a successful skincare regimen that will transform your complexion.

The Actual Role of Moisturizers: Explore the vital role that moisturisers play in maintaining healthy, hydrated skin. Learn how to choose the right moisturiser for your skin type and discover tips for maximising its effectiveness.

The Genuine but Often Underestimated: Sunscreen: Uncover the truth about sunscreen and its crucial role in protecting your skin from the harmful effects of UV radiation. Learn why sunscreen is a non-negotiable step in your skincare routine and how to choose the best sun protection for your needs.

Nourishing Your Skin: Delve into the importance of nourishing your skin from the inside out. Explore the role of nutrition, hydration, and lifestyle factors in promoting radiant, healthy skin and discover simple strategies for enhancing your skin's vitality.

Special Care for Everyone: Serums and Spot Treatment: Unlock the power of targeted skincare solutions with serums and spot treatments. Learn how these potent formulations can address specific concerns such as hydration, brightening, and anti-aging, and discover how to incorporate them into your daily routine for maximum results.

Embracing All Shades: Black Skin Care: Celebrate the beauty and diversity of black skin with tailored skincare tips and recommendations. Explore the unique needs of melanin-rich skin and learn how to care for and enhance its natural radiance.

Important Skincare Anti-aging Ingredients: Discover the key ingredients that can help combat the signs of aging and promote youthful, vibrant skin. From retinol and vitamin C to peptides and antioxidants, explore the powerhouse ingredients that belong in your anti-aging arsenal.

Exfoliation: Learn about the benefits of exfoliation and how to incorporate this essential step into your skincare routine. Discover the different types of exfoliants, from physical scrubs to chemical peels, and uncover the secrets to smoother, brighter skin.

As you journey through each chapter of this book, I encourage you to approach the content with an open mind and a willingness to experiment with new techniques and products. Take the time to customise your skincare routine to fit your unique needs and preferences, and remember to enjoy the process of nurturing and caring for your skin.

Here's to radiant, glowing skin and a newfound sense of confidence and self-love!

Chapter 1: Know Your Skin

Understanding your skin type and selecting the most appropriate skincare routine that is tailored to your requirements is the first step toward achieving beautiful skin. The majority of individuals do not have a clear understanding of their skin type, and as a result, they make use of the incorrect kinds of skin care products. To provide just one example, the care that is required to treat dry skin is considerably different from the care that is required to treat oily skin. When treating the incorrect kind of skin, you run the risk of causing irritation, breakouts, and accelerated aging of the skin. To get the most young, healthy, and radiant appearance possible for your skin, it is vital to choose the appropriate skin care regimen that is tailored to your specific skin type.

Understanding Your Unique Glow

There are five major varieties of skin, as described by the American Academy of Dermatology (AAD): oily skin, dry skin, normal skin, combination skin, and sensitive skin.1. There are a variety of traits and requirements that are specific to each skin type, and they may have an impact on the appearance and texture of your complexion. You may begin to make educated choices about your skin by first determining the kind of skin you have. This will allow you to provide your skin with the individualized care and protection it needs both now and in the years to come. So, If you're not sure what your skin type is, keep reading.

Finding your skin type

Your skin type is dependent on the quantity of sebum (oil) your skin generates. Skin's oiliness may alter over time and may also be impacted by variables such as stress, heredity, hormones, humidity, and the natural aging process.

Once you know what to look for, using the common traits mentioned below, pinpointing your skin type can typically be discovered via easy observation.

There are two tests you can run at home to help you understand what sort of skin you have in about 30 minutes: the blotting sheet approach and the "watch and wait" method.

As your body's biggest organ, your skin performs a range of critical and complicated functions, from controlling your body temperature to defending against pathogens. This is particularly true of your skin's outermost layer, generally known as the skin barrier. Composed largely of lipids (such as ceramides), this protective barrier works as the principal gatekeeper between your skin and the external environment, keeping water in and hazardous things out.

Although a healthy skin barrier is vital for all skin types, it's also crucial to recognize that each individual's skin is unique in many ways. This implies that there's no "one size fits all" strategy to creating glowing, healthy-looking skin. However, there are several unifying traits to look for that might help you identify what skin type you have.

Here are the primary factors to bear in mind while determining whether your skin is generally oily, dry, normal, mixed, or sensitive.

Oily Skin: Oily skin generates an overabundance of sebum that causes the skin to look glossy and feel greasy, especially in the T-zone (forehead, nose, and chin). People with oily skin may likely have fewer wrinkles, according to the American Academy of Dermatology (AAD) but they may also be more prone to enlarged pores, acne breakouts, blackheads, and whiteheads.

Keep in mind that just while oily skin generates more natural oils, this doesn't imply that it needs any less moisture than other skin types. Supporting oily skin comes down to picking the correct products that feed and moisturise, without clogging your pores or causing outbreaks. The optimal oily skin regimen should comprise a mild, foamy cleanser that efficiently eliminates debris, excess oil, and other pollutants. It should also contain a lightweight, oil-free, and non-comedogenic moisturiser that offers your oily skin the critical moisture it needs.

Dry Skin: Dry skin often generates fewer natural oils than other kinds of skin. This may cause it to seem dull and become rough, flaky, or even scaly. It frequently feels tight or less elastic, notably dehydrated, and may be prone to displaying more noticeable small wrinkles. In addition, it may become uncomfortable or irritating.

A skincare regimen for dry skin should contain mild, calming, and moisturising components that help maintain the skin's protective moisture barrier—such as ceramides.

Normal Skin: Normal skin is balanced—feeling neither too dry nor overly oily. It is not prone to breakouts, flakiness, or feeling oily or tight. People with normal skin often have tiny pores, and a smooth skin texture, and are less prone to irritation or blemishes. However, even though normal skin doesn't have any special disorders or worries, it still needs basic treatment to look and feel its best. The optimum normal skin regimen helps maintain your skin's hydration by locking in moisture and strengthening your skin's protective barrier.

Combination Skin: Combination skin comprises parts that are dry as well as oily, with the T-zone frequently being oily, and the cheekbones being either dry or normal. This skin type may fluctuate over different seasons of the year, and owing to numerous reasons, such as stress or hormone fluctuation. Effective washing and hydration are crucial to care for skin that's oily or normal in some spots and dry in others.

Sensitive skin: Sensitive skin is commonly referred to as a skin type, although it's possible to have oily sensitive skin, dry sensitive skin, or normal sensitive skin. Regardless matter the kind of skin you have, if you have sensitive skin, it may seem red and feel like it's burning, itchy, or dry. These symptoms may be connected to having skin that is more reactive to external irritants and may be caused by particular ingredients, like dyes or fragrances, as well as environmental variables.

If you have sensitive skin, you may be able to discover what causes your sensitivity and avoid cleansers, moisturisers, or other products containing those exact chemicals. You may also adjust your surroundings to decrease your exposure to triggering chemicals.

Home Methods to Identifying Your Skin Type: Step-by-step Guide

If explanations of the various skin kinds didn't help you come to a decision, there are several tests you can take at home to help you discover your skin type.
Here are two techniques you may use:

The "watch and wait" strategy: This at-home test helps you to learn your skin type by seeing how your skin responds after cleaning.

- To start, wash your face with a light cleanser, then gently pat it dry.
- Wait 30 minutes.
- If your skin seems glossy overall, you likely have oily skin.
- If it feels tight and is flaky or scaly, you likely have dry skin.

- If the shine is just in your T-zone, you probably have combination skin.
- If your skin feels moisturised and comfortable, but not greasy, you likely have normal skin.

The blotting sheet technique: When rubbed to the skin, blotting sheets absorb oil, and you may use them to help you understand what sort of skin you have.

- After washing your face with a light cleanser, pat it dry and wait for 30 minutes.
- Press blotting sheets to different places on your face, then hold the sheets up to the light to see the oil marks.
- If the sheets soak up a lot of oil from all parts of the face, you have oily skin.
- If they absorb little to no oil, then you probably have dry skin.
- If the sheets indicate just a modest quantity of oil from your T-zone, you have mixed skin.

- If you only observe minor oil from every part of your face, you most likely have normal skin.

It's crucial to realise that any skin type may also be sensitive or prone to acne outbreaks, though individuals with normal skin may be less likely to suffer either. However, with the correct solutions, you can care for your skin while addressing problems like irritation and acne breakouts. When in doubt, consult a board-certified dermatologist for a customised skin examination and advice on the ideal skincare regimen for your skin type.

Chapter 2: Building Your Basics

Among humans, cleansing has progressed a long way beyond dirt removal. It is a ritual done by man from the time of his inception and has been an integral aspect of religious ceremonial and beliefs. In modern times, the process of cleaning to many individuals serves as a form of relaxation and escape from the vicissitudes of regular life, and also as a technique to enhance skin health and attractiveness. Irrespective of the viewpoint, a careful balance has to be maintained between skin washing and the maintenance of its homeostatic capabilities.

Whilst we increasingly utilise skincare products on our skin, we appear to be leaving out or performing a rush job of the most fundamental and crucial component of our beauty routine: cleaning. But a fast sweep of a face wipe or spraying your face with water in the shower won't cut it. Taking the time to remove your makeup and properly wash your face will guarantee that you notice obvious results day after day, cleanse after cleanse.

Hygiene is the practice of keeping oneself and one's surroundings clean to avoid sickness or disease. Consequently, skin hygiene comprises both skin washing and also taking care of its health.

Why you need cleansers

Many of the environmental contaminants and cosmetic items are not water soluble and therefore bathing the skin with simply water would not be adequate to eliminate them. Substances capable of emulsifying them into finer particles are to be utilised for rendering these fat-soluble contaminants water-soluble. Herein, cleansers fit into the picture. Skin cleansers are surface active chemicals (i.e. emulsifiers/detergents/surfactants/soaps) that reduce the surface tension on the skin and remove dirt, sebum, and oil from cosmetic products, germs, and exfoliated corneum cells in an emulsified state. An excellent cleanser should achieve all this without hurting or irritating the skin, on the contrary, it should aim to maintain the skin surface wet.

The Importance of Gentle Skin Cleansing for Everyone: Nurturing Your Complexion for Optimal Health

A regular skincare regimen is vital for preserving a bright complexion. Among its primary processes, cleaning serves a crucial function in eliminating impurities, excess oil, and environmental toxins that collect on the skin's surface. However, the manner and materials used for washing may considerably affect the skin's health and look. By implementing gentle washing procedures, you may nourish your skin and obtain a healthy, beautiful complexion.

Gentle skin cleaning is vital for preserving the skin's natural balance while successfully eliminating contaminants. Harsh soaps or cleansers containing aggressive substances may take away the skin's protective oils, upset its pH balance, and damage its barrier function. This may result in dryness, inflammation, and a variety of skin issues. By using a moderate, pH-balanced cleanser, you may wash your skin without causing undue harm or disturbance.

Consider what your skin is exposed to during the day. From makeup and perspiration to particles in the environment, your skin unavoidably meets several external aggressors. Daily facial cleaning eliminates every last trace of debris, excess oil, pollutants and undesirable skin cells off of your face.

Cleansing is the initial step of all skincare regimes and is useful in a variety of ways. If not washed correctly, grime and impurities gather at the surface of your skin and might lead to breakouts, dehydration, and ageing.

There are various advantages to utilising a cleanser, not only for your face. Cleansers might help you feel more awake, focused, and remain fresh.
Here are several advantages of utilising a cleaner.

Maintain a clean skin: To help defend itself from environmental harm, the skin generates sebum. While sebum is helpful to your skin, if it lingers on the skin too long without being wiped off, or if there is enough oil on the surface, it may combine with any remaining build-up still on your skin. This may produce enlarged pores and create a blockage of skin follicles, trapping sebum and enabling germs to enter the skin, which leads to irritation, acne, and a blotchy and lackluster complexion.

Boost hydration: Regular face cleaning is also a key aspect in helping the skin retain a suitable amount of moisture. Dehydrated skin looks and feels rough, wrinkled, and aged. Cleansing helps control the pH levels of the skin; permitting appropriate water and product retention, for optimal skin hydration.

Stay young-looking: Every day, your skin is aging. Pollution and environmental pollutants may accelerate the ageing process, and the relatively easy procedure of washing your skin is a fantastic approach to getting rid of any undesirable particles and activating the internal processes, which combat ageing, including wrinkles, loss of tone, pigmentation, and dullness.

Increase product's effectiveness: Without washing, your skin would be coated with a thick layer of filth and grime which would make it impossible for the active substances placed over to reach the skin correctly and therefore operate. Clearing up your pores will prepare your skin for the absorption of other skincare products and will thus make it more susceptible to treatments to follow such as exfoliators, masks, serums, and moisturisers, for optimal efficacy.

Reduce the appearance of fine lines and wrinkles.
Cleansers that include exfoliating beads may also help to minimise the appearance of fine lines and wrinkles. The beads operate by sloughing off dead skin cells, exposing the brighter, smoother skin underlying. In addition, cleansers that include antioxidants may help to protect the skin from damage caused by free radicals. As a consequence, utilising a cleanser targeted to your unique skincare requirements may help lessen the look of fine lines and wrinkles.

Reduce redness and inflammation: Skin cleansers may assist in decreasing redness and irritation by eliminating dirt, debris, and makeup from the skin. Look for cleansers that include aloe vera, chamomile, and green tea to help soothe the skin. Avoid cleansers with strong chemicals or perfumes, since they may further irritate the skin.

Boost immunological system: Most people think of cleansers to erase dirt, makeup, and other unpleasant items on their skin. However, did you know that they may also enhance your immune system?

Cleansers function by eliminating germs and other pollutants from the skin. This leaves your skin healthy and free from illness. In addition, it also helps to eliminate any hazardous poisons that may have built up over time.

The usage of cleansers might assist in maintaining your immune system working at its optimum. Keeping your skin clean and healthy makes you less likely to become ill or get infections. Using a decent-quality cleanser may be just as essential as taking care of your food and getting enough exercise. So next time you're shopping for a new skincare product, don't forget to check out the cleansers!

Improves digestion: Most individuals recognize that strong digestion is vital to overall health but may not know how cleaning might aid improve digestion. Cleansing helps eliminate impurities from the body, resulting to increased absorption of nutrients, improved excretion, and a stronger immune system. In addition, cleaning aids the body's natural detoxification process, which helps sweep out toxic substances that might damage cells and lead to illness.

Choosing the Right Cleanser

When picking a cleanser, aim for one that is created precisely for your skin type. Different cleansers cater to varied requirements, such as oily or acne-prone skin, dry or sensitive skin, or combination skin. Look for cleansers that are marketed as "gentle," "mild," or "non-comedogenic," since they are less likely to cause irritation or clog pores.

pH-Balanced Cleansing

The skin's natural pH is somewhat acidic, often ranging between 4.5 and 5.5. This pH balance helps maintain the skin's protective barrier and provides a healthy habitat for beneficial bacteria. Using pH-balanced cleansers helps ensure that the skin's acid layer is kept, enabling it to operate efficiently. Cleansers having a pH comparable to that of the skin assist avoid over-drying, maintain moisture levels, and enhance overall skin health.

Establishing a Healthy Cleansing Routine

To get the most out of your cleaning process, follow these practical tips:

Frequency: Cleanse your face twice a day, once in the morning and once in the evening. This regular washing procedure helps eliminate pollutants acquired during the day and throughout the night.

Gentle Application: When washing, use your fingers or a soft, clean towel to gently massage the cleanser onto your skin. Avoid using aggressive scrubbing strokes, since they might irritate the skin.

Avoid Hot Water: While it may be tempting, avoid using hot water to wash your face. Hot water may strip the skin of its natural oils and produce dryness. Instead, use lukewarm water to preserve the skin's hydration.

Makeup Removal: Before cleaning, ensure that all makeup is properly removed. Leaving makeup on overnight may clog pores, lead to breakouts, and impair the skin's natural regeneration process.

Pat Dry: After cleansing your face, gently pat it dry with a soft cloth. Avoid touching the skin forcefully, since this might create irritation.

Use of cleansers in different dermatologic illnesses

For normal skin, selecting a specific cleanser is less crucial as opposed to persons with dermatological problems such as atopic dermatitis, acne vulgaris, rosacea, photoaging, occupational dermatosis, perianal pruritus, and sensitive skin. In all these circumstances, a cleaning agent that may be used simultaneously with topical treatments and also is biocompatible with the skin condition should be advised.

Cleansing in atopic dermatitis: Atopic dermatitis (AD) occurs as a consequence of a complex interaction of environmental, immunologic, genetic, and pharmaceutical variables. Several trigger factors such as irritants (soap and detergents, occupational irritants, and disinfectants), germs (Staphylococcus aureus, viruses, and dermatophytes), aeroallergens, seasonal changes, and psychogenic factors may worsen the illness. Although most doctors agree that the skin of patients with atopic dermatitis should be maintained clean, there is no consensus of viewpoints about the use of conventional toilet soaps for washing the skin in the course of care for this illness. Washing twice daily with a typical alkaline soap (pH 10.2) was demonstrated to diminish the stratum corneum cell layer and induced attrition of intercellular lipids in patients suffering from atopic dermatitis. This impairment to the epidermal barrier function might result in increased colonization of gram-positive bacteria.

Since soaps have an irritating impact on the skin and AD patients often display a lowered irritation threshold, thus, synthetic washing bars are an excellent alternative for cleaning these individuals. Their mildness and capacity to maintain optimum hydration of the stratum corneum are a gift for atopic dry skin.

Cleansing in acne: The purpose of cleansing for acne or acne-prone skin is to gently remove surface debris, perspiration, and excessive skin lipids without irritating or drying the skin. The perfect cleanser for acne skin should be: non comedogenic, non-acnegenic, nonirritant, and nonallergic

The belief connected with acne is that rigorous washing of the face with soap and water many times a day can decrease the oiliness; nevertheless, simply leads to an exacerbation of acne and occasionally even may produce acne detergents.

There is a broad range of skin cleaning products for acne-prone individuals ranging from lipid-free cleansers, syndets, astringents, exfoliants, and abrasives. The principal adverse effects of most anti-acne therapy are dryness and irritation of the skin, thus gentle cleaning is crucial in this group of patients. A nonionic, fragrance-free dermatologic bar or liquid cleanser with high instability is the best cleanser for acne. The cleaning routine should meet the demands of the particular patient.

Cleansing in rosacea: The skin of people with rosacea is very sensitive to chemical irritants. It is recommended to avoid traditional soaps, and cleansers containing alcohol, astringents, and abrasives in these people. Ideally, only extremely light cleaning products should be utilised in these individuals. If more irritating washing products are employed they should be diluted considerably.

Therapeutic skin cleansers, comprising sulfacetamide 10% and sulphur 5% in addition to a synthetic detergent, are recommended for the treatment of rosacea. Vigorous scrubbing should nonetheless be avoided. The sole contraindication to their usage is known hypersensitivity to sulfonamides, sulphur, or other components. Gentle washing is advised in rosacea sufferers.

Cleansing in photoaged skin: Excessive long-term exposure to sunlight damages the skin, and is believed to promote premature ageing and skin cancer. Since these folks have an already damaged skin surface, thus lipid-free cleaning solutions including humectants and emollients also may aid in lessening the severity of some of the symptoms associated with photoaged skin.

Cleansing in occupational dermatosis: Occupational dermatosis is an important category of conditions seen in practice. Among them, contact dermatitis, both irritating and allergic, is of specific concern. Prevention is the key to lowering the incidence and prevalence of both kinds of contact dermatitis. Avoidance of causative irritants both at home and the workplace is the basic therapy of contact dermatitis. People suffering from these illnesses should adopt proper skin care regularly. Skin washing solutions are equally vital both as skin protection and skin care products in an industrial setting for the removal of soiling. Skin-compatible hand cleaning is crucial for the prevention of occupational dermatitis. The basic requirements for an efficient skin cleanser to prevent occupational skin diseases are its easy solubility in both hard and soft water, its ability to remove fats, oils, and greasy materials without drying the skin, its free flow through the dispensers, and a long shelf life without easy deterioration on storage.

In truth, however, no cleanser can be described as perfect for occupational dermatosis. While liquid synthetic detergents are often completely suitable for washing hands at home, more strong hand cleansers are required for the removal of heavy-duty industrial ceilings such as oil, grease, paints, and lacquer. Products devoid of scrubbing agents are typically skin-friendly and praised by dermatologists.

Cleansing in xerotic skin: Xerotic skin is present in numerous dermatological conditions and also in the elderly population as a component of normal ageing owing to reduced sebum production. Environmental conditions, such as low humidity and wind may further worsen dryness. To rehydrate and soften xerotic skin, emollients, humectants, or keratin-softening agents should be used liberally—immediately after bathing and reapplied as frequently as required to soften xerotic skin and rehydrate it. People with xerosis should utilise washing methods that do not promote more dryness and preferably include humectants and/or emollient substances.

Cleansing in "sensitive skin": Dermatologists and cosmetic scientists describe "sensitive skin" as that which shows contact irritating or allergic responses more easily than the typical population.

This greater response to external influences might be attributed to physiologic phenomena, heightened neurosensory input, higher immunological responsiveness, and/ or compromised barrier function. It is advised that those who have sensitive skin should use extremely light washing solutions. Liquid face cleansers are incredibly efficient and excellent for sensitive skin. These may also be utilised synergistically with topical or systemic treatment.

Cleansing in retinoid-induced dermatitis and post-chemical peel cleansing-induced sensitive skin:

Topical retinoids used in a broad range of dermatological conditions enhance skin sensitivity to irritation. In these circumstances, the patient should use a cleaner that does not worsen the status of their impaired barrier. The humectants and emollients present in lipid-free cleansers might help decrease the symptoms of certain illnesses.

Facial chemical peels are increasingly becoming popular as cosmetic treatments for the treatment of photoaging, wrinkles, scars, and discoloration. Peeling provides controlled harm to the skin that stimulates the development of new skin with an enhanced look. Since the skin is fragile during the surgery and the ensuing time of epithelium regeneration, moderate cleaning products need to be used to minimise adverse responses.

Cleansing in idiopathic perianal pruritus: Perianal pruritus is characterised as an uncomfortable cutaneous feeling that involves scratching of the skin around the anal opening. It might be primary or idiopathic when no obvious cause can be detected or secondary owing to a recognized etiology. Topical corticosteroids are highly successful in managing idiopathic perianal pruritus, but long-term usage might induce atrophy of the skin of the anogenital region. Perianal washing with light liquid cleansers containing humectants may be a safe starting step for decreasing perianal irritation and can be as effective as topical corticosteroids.

Chapter 3: The actual role of moisturisers.

Daily moisturising is crucial for good skin, however, some view it as an aesthetically inclined practice. Our skin is the body's biggest organ and needs constant maintenance to remain youthful, blemish-free, and healthy.

Moisturisers have long been a staple of skin care practices. They have been demonstrated to enhance the water content in the stratum corneum, the skin's outermost layer, which improves dryness.

Do I need to moisturise?

Even while your body has its natural lubricating system of glands that create oil (or sebum) to maintain a protective covering against harsh outside conditions and infections, most of us do require additional hydration following the devastation that sun, weather, and harsh chemicals wreak on our skin.

Certain persons cannot genetically keep the top layer of skin intact and lack the required lipids to seal in moisture. Some drugs (particularly cholesterol-lowering agents and isotretinoin) may also impact the skin's ability to appropriately retain moisture. If you chance to be one of such persons you might benefit from a daily moisturiser.

Even persons with oily skin may require moisturisers if they peel their natural protective layer with harsh cleansers. However, persons with normal to oily skin who are not exposed to severe external circumstances and/or products and can create enough sebum to protect the skin do not necessarily require extra moisture and are better off investing in an antioxidant serum.

Choosing the Right Moisturiser for Your Skin

There are face creams, body and facial moisturisers, and lotions or ointments for dry, oily, combination, or sensitive skin. Add in anti-aging chemicals and sunscreens and the confusion simply deepens.

So how can you know what moisturiser is best for you? Use these no-nonsense tactics from leading doctors to help pick the appropriate moisturiser for giving your skin the healthy shine you want.

Cream, Lotion, or Ointment?

Picking a moisturiser is a requirement, no matter what sort of skin you have -- oily, dry, or a mix of both.

If you've got itchy or dry skin, you'll probably want to seal in moisture using a thick ointment. Any moisturiser containing alcohols or scents should also typically be avoided for persons with dry skin, since they may make the condition worse. Creams are thinner, help moisturise, and are suitable for regular skin. Lotions are the lightest (water is their major constituent) and are a suitable fit for oily skin.

If you have dark skin, dry spots may be more evident if the dry skin seems pale and scaly. Use a heavy moisturiser for such areas. Look for substances such as ceramides, glycerin, castor oil, petroleum jelly, and hemp seed oil.

Base the thickness of your moisturiser on when and where you apply it on your body, select a light moisturiser for the day and a thicker one for sleep. You may also use a heavier cream for your body and a lightweight hydrating lotion for your face. Stick with lighter, moisturising moisturisers throughout the hot months.

Those with sensitive skin may wish to stick to products containing glycerin since the other components might generate a burning sensation on inflamed skin. You should also avoid occlusives in regions that are prone to acne.

Things to Avoid When Choosing a Moisturiser

More isn't necessarily better when it comes to the list of ingredients in a moisturiser. To receive the best advantage for your skin, eliminate these popular additions.

Colorings and scents: Whether you want to hydrate dry skin, sensitive skin, or anything in between, most experts suggest avoiding superfluous and possibly irritating chemicals, such as added colours and perfumes. Antibacterial agents may often be unduly harsh, depriving skin of vital oils.

Too many acids: Avoid alpha-hydroxy acids, glycolic acid, retinoic acid, and salicylic acid if you have dry or sensitive skin. These substances may enter the skin too deeply and upset fragile skin. Stay away from items containing alcohol as well.

Overusing steroidal components (for itchy skin): Limit your usage of steroid cream or ointment to just one or two weeks unless your doctor suggests using it longer. Overusing these lotions might make skin exceedingly thin and lead to additional skin issues.

Body-friendly ingredients: What's excellent for your body isn't necessarily terrific for your face. It's encouraged to avoid face moisturizers containing popular body product components like lanolin, mineral oil, waxes, or shea butter. These may block pores and produce acne on the face.

Urea or Lactic acids (for eczema or cracked skin): Stay clear from moisturisers that include these dry-skin-friendly chemicals. They might worsen existing skin irritations.

Tips to Achieving the Best Results

1. The optimal time to apply a moisturiser is while the skin is still wet. After using a mild cleanser, softly massage your skin wet, and then immediately apply a layer of moisturiser to seal in the moisture. Though a thorough moisturising routine is a terrific start, it is crucial to keep hydrated and receive key nutrients (vitamins, essential fatty acids) that are the building blocks for healthy skin. Avoiding smoking and adopting excellent sun protection are vital for long-term skin care.

2. Use more than one moisturiser (if you need to). Nobody needs a cupboard full of hydrating creams. But a light lotion for your face and a thick cream for your body may be just suitable for your all-over skin care.

3. Make your moisturiser perform double duty. Want to balance out your skin tone?

Look for a tinted moisturiser fit for your complexion.

Chapter 4: The genuine but often underestimated

The Secret to Ageless Skin: Sunscreen

The purpose of any sunscreen is to help shield your skin from injury caused by exposure to the sun, and a broad-spectrum product that helps protect against UVA and UVB rays is necessary for all skin types and ethnicities, including yours. Sun protection is vital while spending longer amounts of time outside; but, it should also be used every morning to help avoid cumulative damage caused by shorter exposure intervals and indirect sunlight (such as when driving or going to and from your vehicle). Available in lotion, cream, stick, and other formulas suited for newborns, children, and adults, no matter what your age or lifestyle, there's an effective wide-spectrum sun protection product for you. But the key to gaining the advantages of sunscreen and preserving healthy skin is using it as advised.

How sunscreen really works

Sunscreen solutions are meant to help prevent sunburn, and broad-spectrum protection is vital to help shield your skin from UVA and UVB radiation. When UV rays reach the skin, they disturb your cells' regular development and function, and they tear down your skin's collagen and elastin (which leads to lines and wrinkles).

Sunscreens function in one of two ways, depending on the UV filter chemicals in your sun protection solution. Sunscreens containing chemical-based components, such as homosalate, operate by penetrating the top layers of your skin and absorbing UV rays before they can harm your skin cells. Mineral (sometimes called physical) sun filters, including zinc oxide and titanium dioxide, form a barrier on your skin's surface that bounces UV radiation off the skin. Some sun protection solutions feature a combination of both chemical and mineral sun filters.

Importance of Sunscreen for all Skin Tones.

Applying sunscreen every day should be the core of your skin care regimen. You probably know some of the reasons why sunscreen is so essential, but others of them may be new to you. Here are several reasons why you should use sunscreen.

Prevents Premature Aging: All of us wish to have younger-looking, beautiful, and healthy skin. This is one of the most persuasive reasons to start wearing sunscreen. Indulging in outdoor activities without sufficient sun protection may exacerbate indications of aging. Prevention is crucial and is feasible with the aid of sunscreen application. It defends your skin from acquiring indications of aging, such as wrinkles and fine lines, sunspots, hyperpigmentation, photodamagei, (sun damage), and dry skin. Studies indicate that those below the age of 55 who used sunscreen had a 24% lower likelihood of getting these aging indicators than non-sunscreen and occasional sunscreen users.

Shields From damaging UV Rays: The continually diminishing ozone layer has placed us at a larger risk of being impacted by the damaging rays of the sun. While you need the sun for your daily dosage of Vitamin D, it does not mean that you should put your health in danger! This radiation may lead to sunburn and skin damage. Sunscreens are vital goods that protect you from dangerous UV radiation.

Lowers Skin Cancer Risk: While individuals began wearing sunscreen largely for appearance reasons, this health benefit comes as an upside.

Wear your sunscreen regularly and throughout the days and months to guard your skin from the danger of numerous forms of skin cancer. This is the deadliest sort of skin cancer, which may be life-threatening for women as their age grows.

Enhances Health Of The Skin: The vital skin proteins, such as collagen, keratin, and elastin, are protected by sunscreen. These proteins are necessary for keeping the skin smooth and healthy. Make sure your sunscreen includes titanium dioxide in it to help scatter UV rays away from the skin and safeguard the action of these proteins.

Prevents Sunburns: Sunburns may thin the skin, making it more translucent, and bruises become more evident. Your skin may undergo recurring outbreaks of peeling, swelling, redness, hives, and itching. This is due to UVB radiation, responsible for sunburns. The blisters might enhance the risk of skin cancer.

It helps maintain even skin tone: Sun spots and uneven skin tone are usually caused by sun exposure. Even if you are taking retinol for anti-aging, they will not stop the sunspots or discolorations occurring if you're not also protecting your skin with sunscreen.

Exfoliated skin burns easier: If you're using skin care products containing alpha hydroxy acids (AHAs), your skin will be more susceptible to UV radiation and sunscreen is even more vital. And this is still the case even if you just use these products at night, your skin will still be sensitive the following day and for some time thereafter.

So if you have acids that figure in your regimen, it's extremely crucial to make sure you're safeguarding your lovely skin by wearing sunscreen.

You May Not Have To Reapply After A Swim: Most of the sunscreens or sunblocks available these days are waterproof. This permits you to enjoy yourself in the water, without burning yourself.

Sunscreen Offers Better Protection Than A Full-Sleeved Dress: You cannot defend yourself from the sun by wearing a full-sleeved dress. Did you know that a cotton garment, especially when moist, provides zero protection from the damaging rays of the sun? Just put a good quantity of sunscreen beneath the clothing as well.

How To Choose A Sunscreen For Your Skin Type

Of fact, many sunscreens—both physical and chemical—augment their active components with additional skincare products that might give further advantages for common skin concerns.

For dry skin: It's not too difficult to detect a decent dry-skin moisturizer. Ingredients like ceramides and hyaluronic acid that exist naturally in the skin (and help it execute its barrier function) are also typically present in sunscreens intended for dry skin. A mineral solution with some thickness and moisturizing skincare could be a nice place to start.

For oily skin: Some individuals with oily skin like chemical sunscreen for how it soaks rapidly into the skin; others who lean acne-prone enjoy mineral formulations that aren't as likely to linger in the pores and create outbreaks. There are lots of sunscreen formulations developed for persons with oily skin, both mineral, and chemical, that feature niacinamide, which has two-fold purifying and protective power: It may help decongest pores and prevent the accumulation of oil and debris.

For mature skin: This skin type has an extra motivation for sun protection since the effects of aging are hastened by sun overexposure. Those with mature skin type should pick a sunscreen packed with reparative elements, such as antioxidants, which may help battle cellular damage, including damage caused by photoaging.

For sensitive skin: For sensitive skin SPF, avoid formulations that have additional scents or colors, both of which may be potentially irritating. Dry sensitive skin could react well to hydrating substances that provide skin-soothing properties. A non-comedogenic (read: won't clog pores) solution, on the other hand, is perfect for oily sensitive skin that can be prone to pimples

The Right Way to Use Sunscreen

How to apply sunscreen every day? If you are thinking about it, here are a few aspects and sun safety advice that you need to bear in mind when selecting up the sunscreen:

1. Always examine the ingredient list and make sure your sunscreen has the following:
   - Titanium dioxide
   - Octyl methoxycinnamate (OMC)

- Avobenzonei (also parsol)
- Zinc oxide

2. Opt for a broad-spectrum sunscreen lotion or gel that is non-comedogenic and hypoallergenic. Such sunscreens will shelter you from UV radiation, both A and B, while preserving you against rashes, blocked pores, acne, and sunburns.
3. Choose a sunscreen that is waterproof and comes with a minimum SPF of 30. 4. Always apply sunscreen half an hour before you come into touch with the sun.

How Often You Should Use Sunscreens

Sunscreens work as a guard against the dangerous UV rays that breach the skin's barrier every time your skin is exposed to the sun. It is, therefore, recommended to wear sunscreen every day. You may not feel the advantages today, but the advantage of taking sunscreen is realized in the long term. If you are out in the sun for a long period either working or enjoying a sunbath on the beach or at the poolside, it is best to reapply sunscreen after every two hours to protect your skin from sunburns. Consult a doctor to learn more about sunscreen reapplication intervals .best suited for your skin type.

Possible Concerns about Sunscreen

Photosensitivity: Some persons may develop unpleasant responses owing to specific components that make the skin more sensitive when exposed to the sun, consequently producing sunburn or inflammation.

Skin Irritation: Some persons may be allergic or sensitive to particular compounds found in sunscreens and, consequently, suffer inflammation, itching, and redness.

Acne Breakouts: Some sunscreens include pore-clogging chemicals that may trigger your skin to break out.

Increased Risk Of Cancer: Benzophenone-3 is a chemical included in many sunscreens that has been demonstrated to adversely influence estrogen levels and raise the risk of breast cancer.

Best Sunscreens Suitable for Everyday Use.

Before you go grabbing any sunscreen, it's crucial to realize that they aren't all made equal. So how do you find the appropriate one for you and your family? Take a peek!

Pay Attention To The Active Ingredients: There are two kinds of sunscreens – mineral sunscreen and chemical sunscreen. As you may have suspected, the components in each vary dramatically.

In chemical sunscreen, some of the active chemicals include oxybenzone, octinoxate, octisalate, and avobenzone.

Chemical sunscreen could shield you from the damaging rays of the sun, but that comes at a cost for both you and the environment!

The chemicals in the sunscreen may permeate your skin and ultimately enter your system.

On the other hand, mineral sunscreen is manufactured from just two active ingredients—zinc oxide and titanium dioxide. These minerals remain on the surface of your skin and don't permeate it.

Some of the alternatives accessible to you will be explored, but for now, it's only necessary to understand that going for mineral sunscreen is excellent for both your skin and the environment.

Look At The SPF: Sun Protection Factor (SPF) is a measure of how effectively your sunscreen will protect you from the UV and UV radiation of the sun. These rays are renowned for causing sunburn, premature skin ageing, and leading to skin cancer.

When you use daily sunscreen, the sun protection must contain the proper quantity of SPF for you and your requirements.

But what number should you be searching for?

The American Academy of Dermatology stresses that, "Dermatologists recommend using a sunscreen with an SPF of at least 30, which blocks 97 percent of the sun's UV rays. Higher number SPFs block somewhat more of the sun's UV rays, but no sunscreen can block 100 percent of the sun's UV rays."

While on this issue, it's crucial to stress that applying a product with a higher SPF doesn't indicate that it will last longer. You still need to reapply the sunscreen every couple of hours to ensure that you continue obtaining enough protection.

Make Sure It's Gentle On Skin: As we discussed before, some sunscreen creams are laden with loads of toxic components. These chemicals might end up blocking your pores and can cause inflammation.
You need a product that will be effective without damaging you! But it should also have hydrating characteristics and be gentle on your skin.

Chapter 5: Nourishing Your Skin

Smart eating choices are smart investments. Eating the proper quantity of nourished food via a balanced diet has been recognized to offer many health advantages. Therefore, it should come as no surprise that the secret to attaining bright, vibrant skin is also consuming good food. After all, only skin that is healthy from the inside shines from the outside.

The thought is that during the day our skin is prone to environmental wear and tear and the ingestion of junk food that naturally messes with the process of skin cell turnover and the ability to retain more moisture in our skin. Therefore, our skin ends up appearing more drab and dry. However, obtaining the correct meal may alter that.

Feeding your Skin from within

Our skin has numerous layers and structures which change throughout time. This is perfectly normal and might include acne, pigmentation, wrinkles, or sagging. The amount to which these structures emerge is controlled by both internal (endogenous) and external (exogenous) variables.

The capacity of plants to enhance skin health is encouraging since they may help decrease inflammation, strengthen skin structures, and guard against harm. Enjoying a range of good meals is beneficial for the body, including our skin. Let's investigate this further.

<u>Tips to nourish skin from within</u>

Add in bright fruits and vegetables: Fruits and vegetables give a plethora of nutrients and antioxidants that maintain our skin, particularly when we eat a diversity of hues. Enjoying fruits and vegetables, which are great sources of antioxidants, has been related to good effects on skin elasticity, wrinkling, roughness, and color. Consider eating a vivid and bright selection of fruits and vegetables as pleasantly sweet sources of antioxidants. For example, some fruits and vegetables especially high in antioxidants include:

- Bell peppers.
- Citrus fruits.
- Dark leafy greens.
- Grapes.
- Mangoes.
- Passion fruit.
- Pomegranate.

Hold onto Hydration: The skin's capacity to resist excess water loss is vital. Some kinds of fats, such as omega-3 fats, seem to have the ability to increase skin barrier function which may help hold onto water. Due to its anti-inflammatory effects, obtaining adequate omega-3 fats is also promising for illnesses such as dermatitis, psoriasis, and acne.

Hydration also plays a crucial part in the health of our skin, and having enough water has been related to less dry and rough skin in individuals not currently drinking enough. It's been advised that at least 2 litres every day has advantages for skin health, and this may include simple water on its own, or in fluids found in soups, fruits, smoothies, and teas. Some indicators that we're insufficiently hydrated include feeling thirsty, having dry skin or lips, and dark yellow urine.

Some additional reasons that may contribute to dry skin include weather, the use of certain skin creams, and excessive sun exposure. Sometimes, our skin might even stay dry without environmental variables at play owing to skin diseases such as eczema. In these circumstances, the underlying problems must be initially treated, however, nutrition may occasionally give further help.

Embrace plant proteins from meals first: Protein makes up a big component of our skin, and this makes it a critical role in keeping our skin robust and healthy. Key proteins that promote smooth and robust skin include elastin, collagen, and keratins.

When we ingest protein, it's broken down into smaller building blocks called amino acids, and our body utilizes these smaller units to produce proteins where they're required. This means if we take a collagen protein supplement, for example, it will be broken down into smaller parts (amino acids or peptides) to construct proteins throughout the body. This may or may not involve the skin. So instead of depending on supplements, we might consider adopting a foods-first approach.

Plant foods high in protein include a broad range of legumes, cereals, vegetables, nuts, and seeds. Getting adequate protein overall makes sure we have the building blocks for our skin's critical structures.

Interestingly, dietary patterns rich in animal items such as dairy and meat have also been related to an increase in acne probably owing to growth and sex hormones that may induce inflammation in the body. Plant-based protein sources nevertheless, such as legumes and nuts, have been related to reduced levels of inflammation.

Consider slower digesting carbohydrates: Some meals break down into sugar in the body faster than others which may increase inflammation, acne, or hasten symptoms of aging with excess consumption. Carbohydrates that break down into sugar fast are considered high glycemic, such as sugar-sweetened drinks, refined grains, or sweets. Since these meals break down into sugar quicker, the quantity of sugar in the blood also rises quickly. This boosts hormone levels, such as insulin and insulin-like growth factors, which may drive increased sebum (oil) production and acne. Foods that transform into sugar gradually, such as whole grains are considered low glycemic and have shown favorable effects on the skin.

Another problem is that broken-down sugar, such as glucose, may mix with protein in the skin, such as collagen, to generate what's called advanced glycation end products or "AGEs". AGEs may increase inflammation and stress which may damage skin health. High blood sugar levels may increase AGEs, in addition to meals rich in them such as fried foods, high-fat spreads, and oils.

In brief, you may consider consuming a range of healthful plant foods like fruits, vegetables, legumes, grains, nuts, and seeds, and minimize overly processed meals with added sugars and oils whenever feasible. To investigate sugar more explicitly, visit our page with methods to limit additional sugars.

Keep the stomach happy: Our skin provides a useful insight into what's going on within the body and an expanding topic of research in the effect of gut health on skin. When we ingest food, broken-down particles finally reach the big intestine, where millions of microorganisms reside, such as bacteria. This undigested food may feed the microbes, enabling their development, and in turn, generate a small ecosystem in the gut. It's suggested the kinds and number of bacteria in our gut ecology may be associated with skin health. For example, an increase in disease-promoting bacteria in the stomach has been connected with acne. Foods that feed good microbes are termed prebiotics such as fiber-rich whole grains, beans, bananas, and cruciferous vegetables. Whereas probiotics supply the live microbes themselves.

Probiotics are prospective actors in the prevention and treatment of skin disorders such as acne and eczema. They may minimize breakouts via favorable effects on inflammation and sebum production. While more study is required for a deeper understanding, consuming fermented foods such as kombucha, kimchi, sauerkraut, miso, or sourdough bread may give probiotics and are a wonderful choice to help support our gut-skin axis.

Cut down on alcohol: Consuming alcohol has the potential to damage skin health since it may diminish vitamin A status in the skin or hydration.

Some alternative drinks to alcohol to consider include:

- Flavoring water with antioxidant-rich fruit, vegetables, or herbs.
- Blending up a smoothie.
- Refreshing with a source of wonderful probiotics, kombucha.

Nutrients and skin health

Enjoying a broad range of plant-based meals boosts general health, and several nutrients are well renowned for their skin health-boosting potential.

You may consider the following nutrients and sources.

Nutrient	Benefits	Food Sources
Vitamin A	Essential for the growth and maintenance of healthy skin cells; may protect against skin cancer.	beef liver, sweet potato, spinach, carrots, cantaloupe
Vitamin B2 (Riboflavin)	Helps maintain collagen levels in the skin.	beef liver, fortified breakfast cereals, dairy, mushrooms, almonds
Vitamin B6	Deficiency	chickpeas,

(pyridoxine)	can cause skin rashes, and cracks in the skin around the mouth.	beef liver, poultry, salmon, fortified breakfast cereals, potatoes, bananas
Vitamin C	An antioxidant that helps form the skin barrier and collagen, protects against sun damage, and reduces the risk of some skin diseases.	citrus fruits, bell peppers, kiwi, broccoli, strawberries
Vitamin D	May play a role in wound	cod liver oil, seafood,

	healing, protection against sun damage, and in reducing inflammation.	UV-exposed mushrooms, fortified dairy milk and plant milks, fortified breakfast cereals
Vitamin E	An antioxidant that helps protect against sun damage.	wheat germ oil, sunflower seeds, almonds, sunflower oil, peanut butter
Omega-3 fatty acids	May help some skin conditions and protect against sun damage.	flaxseed oil, chia seeds, walnuts, salmon, herring, mackerel, canola oil

Zinc	Helps skin integrity and wound healing.	oysters, beef, crab, pork, baked beans, fortified breakfast cereals, pumpkin seeds, chickpeas

Chapter 6: Special Care for Everyone

In skin care, personalized care is crucial, and serums and spot treatments are useful tools in addressing specific requirements. These specialist products provide focused treatments developed to satisfy particular skin conditions, guaranteeing that everyone may reach their desired goals.

The Powerhouses of Skincare: Understanding Serums

Serums are strong skincare formulas meant to deliver a high concentration of active ingredients deep into the skin. With their lightweight and fast-absorbing properties, serums can enter the skin more efficiently than other treatments like moisturizers or creams.

In this part, we'll look into the advantages of serums and how they may address common skincare problems including hydration, brightening, and anti-aging.

Revealing the Beauty Benefits of Serums

Hydration: Serums are commonly made with moisturizing substances like hyaluronic acid, glycerin, or ceramides. These humectants attract moisture into the skin, helping to plump and moisturize from the inside.

By supplying a rush of hydration deep into the skin's layers, serums may successfully counteract dryness, tightness, and flakiness, leaving the skin smooth, supple, and radiant.

Brightening and Even-Toning: Many serums include chemicals like vitamin C, niacinamide, or licorice extract, which have brightening characteristics. These chemicals act to remove dark spots, hyperpigmentation, and uneven skin tone, resulting in a more luminous complexion. By blocking melanin synthesis and boosting cell turnover, brightening serums may help reveal smoother, more radiant skin over time.

Anti-Aging and Wrinkle Reduction: Serums loaded with powerful antioxidants like vitamin E, green tea extract, or resveratrol may help fight the skin against environmental damage and free radicals, which contribute to premature aging. Additionally, serums containing peptides, retinol, or growth factors boost collagen formation and cellular turnover, minimizing the appearance of fine lines, wrinkles, and sagging skin.

By increasing firmness, elasticity, and general skin renewal, anti-aging serums may help restore a young, beautiful complexion.

Spot Treatment

Put simply, a spot treatment is a form of concentrated skincare solution meant to assist manage acute skin issues, mainly pimples. They frequently include salicylic acid, benzoyl peroxide, or other blemish-fighting compounds and are supposed to be applied specifically to the problem region rather than all over the face (thus the name). And this isn't the only manner in which they qualify as a targeted therapy. Unlike serums and moisturizers, spot treatments aren't normally designed for everyday usage; instead, they're used as required until the condition passes. While acne spot treatments are far and away the most prevalent sort of spot treatments, you may also discover solutions that target dark spots and discolorations, such as post-blemish marks.

Spot treatment is most typically a cream, gel, serum, or patch used to treat and minimize active acne blemishes and post-acne scars or dark spots. They frequently include high quantities of active chemicals, such as salicylic acid (a beta hydroxy acid) or niacinamide (vitamin B3) to decrease swelling, redness, and irritation. Some creams or gels might produce a tiny film on the skin somewhat like an acne patch. However, a lot of spot treatments are produced from hydrocolloid dressings that aid in minimizing swelling and irritation.

Spot treatments come in many various formulations but their primary purpose is to aid in speeding up the healing process by decreasing inflammation and redness. They also assist in minimizing the look of acne.

There are also spot treatments that help diminish post-acne scars, sun spots, or dark spots. These regimens will commonly contain brightening substances like L-ascorbic acid or retinoids.

How to Use a Spot Treatment

Other spot treatments are applied specifically to blemishes, while others are administered all over the face you always want to cure and avoid. All-over treatments are advised, and then spot treatments if you have anything that breaks through your all-over treatment. An all-over treatment would be a facial serum that's applied to the whole face to help brighten the complexion, while a spot treatment would be a product that's used solely on certain parts of the skin to address issues like dark patches or active breakouts.

Pay attention to the label on your skincare to ensure you're using you're treatment as intended, and always speak with your dermatologist before adding a new product or component to your skin care regimen.

Here's a basic instruction on how to utilize a spot treatment in your skin care regimen.

1. Prepare the Skin: Before using a product or spot treatment, wash your skin. Applying any form of face serum or spot treatment on filthy skin will have terrible efficacy and may even lead to serious discomfort.

2. Apply Your Facial Serums: If you're using a facial serum to tackle particular skin issues, such as dullness, dark spots, or acne outbreaks, apply it all over the skin. Follow the directions in the box for the right application. Products like these try to prevent and treat particular skin issues and are most effective when they're applied to your full face.

3. Apply Your Tailored Spot Treatment: After all-over serums come tailored treatments. The distinction is that a focused treatment is going to be administered specifically to blemishes or dark spots (depending on what you're treating), not all over the face. A spot treatment assists in targeting blemishes that break through your other treatments and face serums.

4. Moisturise: No skin care regimen is complete without moisturiser, regardless of your skin type.

It will assist in locking in moisture so your serums and spot treatments can enter the skin and perform efficiently.

Chapter 7: Embracing All Shades: Black Skin Care

Black skin covers a diversity of tones and textures, each representing a rich ancestry and distinct beauty. Yet, the skincare industry has frequently failed to appropriately meet the various demands of black skin. This section seeks to cast focus on the complexity of black skin, appreciating its intrinsic beauty and pushing for personalized treatment. It will dive into the subtleties of black skin, appreciating its distinctiveness and aiming for inclusiveness.

The Unique Beauty of Black Skin: A Celebration in Skincare

Black skin carries a special and compelling beauty that merits attention and appreciation within the world of skincare. From its high melanin content to its innate resilience, black skin contains distinct traits that set it apart and need specific care.

In this part, we dig into the peculiarities of black skin and stress the significance of appreciating its beauty via mindful skincare methods.

Melanin Magic: Black skin is endowed with copious melanin, the pigment that gives it its deep tone and offers natural protection against the sun's damaging UV rays. This innate sun protection factor (SPF) serves to defend the skin from sun damage, minimizing the risk of sunburn, premature aging, and skin cancer.

While melanin provides built-in protection, it's necessary to supplement this natural defense with a continuous sunscreen program to defend against extended sun exposure and preserve skin health.

Radiant Resilience: Black skin displays a remarkable resilience that enables it to tolerate environmental stimuli and preserve a young look. Its thicker epidermis and greater collagen density contribute to its firmness and elasticity, resulting in less obvious symptoms of aging such as fine lines and wrinkles.

Despite its innate resilience, black skin is not immune to skincare issues such as hyperpigmentation, acne, and dryness. Tailored skincare regimens that suit these particular demands are vital for achieving optimum skin health and brightness.

Hyperpigmentation Harmony:

Hyperpigmentation, marked by dark patches or uneven skin tone, is a frequent skincare problem for those with black skin. Factors such as hormone cycles, sun exposure, and inflammation may worsen hyperpigmentation, resulting in uneven pigmentation and reduced complexion clarity.

Incorporating brightening compounds like vitamin C, niacinamide, and licorice extract into your skincare regimen will help remove dark spots and produce a more even-toned complexion. Additionally, exfoliating chemicals like alpha hydroxy acids (AHAs) and retinoids may accelerate cellular turnover, exposing brighter, more luminous skin over time.

Moisture Mastery: Black skin tends to have greater amounts of natural oils and lipids, resulting in a naturally dewy complexion. However, factors such as severe weather conditions, extensive washing, and low humidity levels may strip the skin of its moisture barrier, resulting in dryness and dehydration.

Hydration is crucial to preserving the health and vibrancy of dark skin. Incorporating hydrating elements like hyaluronic acid, glycerin, and ceramides into your skincare regimen may help replace moisture levels, leaving the skin smooth, supple, and beautiful.

Cultural Connection: Beyond its physical features, black skin contains significant cultural value and acts as a symbol of identity, ancestry, and perseverance. Embracing and expressing the unique beauty of black skin is not just an act of self-love but also a celebration of cultural pride and diversity.

By celebrating the beauty of black skin via skincare techniques that nourish, preserve, and enhance its natural brightness, we affirm its fundamental value and contribute to a more inclusive and representative beauty environment.

Common Skincare Concerns for Black Individuals

Several skin diseases are more frequent or merely seem different on darker skin. Having solid fundamental knowledge would help you take after your skin better.

The extraordinary beauty and richness of melanin-rich skin also come with special concerns. While dark skin gives natural protection from the sun and frequently ages at a slower pace, it's not immune to skin concerns. Let's investigate some of the most prevalent skin issues experienced by black persons and discuss how to manage them successfully.

Hyperpigmentation: Hyperpigmentation is one of the most frequent skin issues among black individuals. It's characterised by black patches or spots that grow owing to increased synthesis of melanin. Factors like sun exposure, acne scars, trauma, hormonal changes, and some medicines may produce hyperpigmentation.

Solutions

1. Sunscreen: Sun exposure may aggravate hyperpigmentation. Daily use of broad-spectrum sunscreen may help avoid this.
2. Topical Treatments: Ingredients including hydroquinone, glycolic acid, and vitamin C help diminish the appearance of black spots.

3. Chemical Peels: Done by specialists, chemical peels may remove the top layers of the skin, minimising the appearance of hyperpigmentation.

Post-Inflammatory Hyperpigmentation (PIH): PIH arises after an injury or inflammation like acne. It shows flat areas of discoloration.

Solutions
1. Avoid Picking: Resist the impulse to pick at places or scars. This may prevent the start of PIH.
2. Topical Retinoids: These may speed cell turnover, helping to minimise the appearance of PIH.
3. Chemical Peels: As indicated, chemical peels may aid in decreasing the appearance of hyperpigmentation.

Keloids: Keloids are elevated scars that expand beyond the initial injury site. They occur because of an overproduction of collagen during the healing process and are more frequent in black persons.

Solutions

1. Pressure Therapy: Applying pressure to a keloid may occasionally diminish its size.
2. Steroid Injections: Administered by a dermatologist, they may help flatten the keloid.
3. Silicone Gel Sheets: These sheets help flatten keloids over time.

Central Centrifugal Cicatricial Alopecia (CCCA): CCCA is a kind of hair loss that normally begins at the crown of the head and progresses outward. It's more frequent in black women and might be caused by things including hairstyle methods and heredity.

Solutions

1. Hair Care: Avoid tight hairstyles and high heat. Instead, go for looser designs and minimum heat exposure.

2. Topical or Oral Treatments: Consulting with a dermatologist may give particular drugs to assist control this disease.

Acne: Acne is a common skin issue which is also sometimes termed pimples or breakouts. It may show at any age on the face, neck, back, and shoulders. They arise when the body's natural oils (sebum) and old skin cells combined restrict the skin's pores. This causes inflammation of the skin.

Solutions

1. Regular Cleansing: Use a mild cleanser to keep pores unclogged.
2. Non-comedogenic Products: Ensure cosmetics and skincare products won't clog pores.
3. Topical therapies: Over-the-counter or prescription therapies help manage and prevent outbreaks.

Dermatosis Papulosa Nigra (DPN): These are little black spots on your face or neck, resembling moles or elevated freckles which typically develop and spread in middle life. They are entirely harmless. DPN is a fairly frequent skin problem among darker-colored Black individuals, women in particular. There are numerous hypotheses on why DPN arises, but the agreement is that it can be treated and eliminated safely.

Solution
Cosmetics won't handle this medical problem. As usual, select a professional aesthetic clinic with vast expertise in treating DPN and managing skin issues in Black skin.

Melanoma: Melanoma is the most dangerous sort of skin cancer. It frequently shows up as a fresh spot on your skin. Or it might be an old area that varies in size, shape, or color. It might even appear like a sore that won't heal or a patch of skin that's rough and dry. If you see any of these skin changes, visit a dermatologist immediately.

It may also show up in locations you would not anticipate, such as your hands and feet. The hands and feet are the most prevalent areas where melanoma is identified in dark-skinned folks. It may also show up below your nails, on the soles of your feet or your palms, or between your fingers and toes.

Solution

Your therapy relies on how deeply the melanoma has grown into your skin and whether it's spread to another region of your body. Your doctor may do surgery to remove the cancer. Other therapies may include T-cell therapy, which harnesses your immune system to attack the malignancy.

Inclusivity in Skincare

Inclusivity in skincare goes beyond simple representation—it's about identifying and embracing the vast variety of skin types, tones, and problems that exist within our communities. It's about providing a place where everyone feels seen, appreciated, and empowered to care for their skin in a manner that acknowledges their individual needs and experiences.

Here is the significance of inclusion in skincare and its influence on people, communities, and the beauty industry as a whole.

Enjoying variety: Inclusivity in skincare embraces the beauty of variety by acknowledging and enjoying the unique qualities of diverse skin types and tones. It recognizes that beauty comes in many hues, textures, and shapes, and attempts to celebrate and promote the vast spectrum of skin identities that exist within our society.

By exhibiting a broad variety of skin tones and types in marketing campaigns, product offers, and brand messaging, skincare firms can reflect the genuine diversity of their customer base and create a more inclusive and representative beauty scene.

Addressing Unmet Needs: Inclusive skincare techniques address the unmet needs of underprivileged populations, including people of colour, persons with sensitive skin, and those with specialised skincare issues such as hyperpigmentation or acne. By delivering products and solutions customised to these requirements, skincare businesses may empower consumers to care for their skin in a manner that promotes health, confidence, and well-being.

For example, formulas targeted to treat hyperpigmentation in darker skin tones, sunscreen alternatives that cater to varied amounts of melanin, and skincare products free from common allergies and irritants may help fulfill the diverse requirements of customers and encourage inclusiveness in skincare.

Fostering Self-Expression and Empowerment: Inclusivity in skincare encourages a feeling of self-expression and empowerment by giving people the skills and resources they need to care for their skin honestly and confidently. It understands that skin care is not only about obtaining a specific appearance but about accepting and enjoying one's unique personality and background.

By providing products that cater to varied skin requirements and concerns, skincare businesses can empower consumers to take control of their skincare journey, experiment with different regimens and formulas, and express themselves authentically via their skincare choices.

Driving Industry Change: Inclusivity in skincare can promote genuine change within the beauty industry by questioning established conventions, standards, and practices that perpetuate exclusion and marginalisation. It demands for increased inclusion and diversity in product development, marketing, and brand leadership, as well as openness and responsibility in advertising and messaging.

By elevating different perspectives, promoting inclusiveness programs, and keeping businesses accountable for their promises to diversity and representation, consumers can drive good change within the skincare industry and build a more inclusive and equitable beauty scene for future generations.

Chapter 8: Important Skincare Anti-aging Ingredients

A variety of components in over-the-counter treatments may make your skin seem more young, but it'll take time. You may experience improvement within a few months. But you shouldn't expect to appear like you've stepped out of a time machine.

What will work best for you depends on your skin and the outcomes you're seeking to attain.

For Wrinkles: Retinol, Vitamin C

If you have fine wrinkles, retinoids (which originate from vitamin A) like retinol may make your face smoother because they help your skin create more collagen. It's softer on your skin than the prescription-strength form, tretinoin (Retin-A), which may dry your skin. Products containing vitamin C may help wipe away fine wrinkles, as well as aid decrease the harm the sun produces to your skin. That might help keep wrinkles away.

For Age Spots: Hydroquinone, Retinoids, Vitamin C, Kojic Acid

Hydroquinone, an over-the-counter medication that may bleach your skin, may erase black spots. Retinoids may make your skin tone more even. One research indicates vitamin C helps reduce age spots when you consume it for 12 weeks. Kojic acid -- a substance that's widely used as a skin-whitening component in goods -- may do that, too.

When you utilise any of them, be sure you apply sunscreen. Your black patches may come back if your skin receives too much sunshine.

For Sagging Skin: Peptides, Ceramides

Treatments with topical growth factors or peptides might help tighten sagging skin. Peptides are groupings of amino acids that help create proteins, including collagen. That's the major protein present in your skin.

Daily moisturisers containing ceramides -- lipids found in the layers of your skin that you lose as you age -- are a choice, too -- and they're generally cheaper.

For Uneven Skin Tone: AHAs, Retinoids

Alpha hydroxy acids (AHAs) destroy dead skin cells. This might assist in disclosing new ones with a more equal tone. Retinoids may achieve the same effect. Both might irritate your skin, so use them with care if yours is dry or sensitive.

For Dull Skin: AHAs, Retinoids

If you smoke or if your skin is dry, you're more likely to have dull skin. A moisturiser may help it seem fuller and firmer. Alpha hydroxy acids

and retinoids (like retinol) might brighten your skin when they eliminate dead skin cells.
Best Anti-aging Skincare Routine Tips

While there is nothing wrong with ageing, who doesn't want to do it gracefully? The easiest approach to do this is to keep healthy and protected skin throughout time
External aggressors such as pollution, stress, and sun exposure enhance the formation of free radicals leading to quicker cellular ageing. In reality, studies reveal that sun radiation, in more than 80% of all instances, is the key contributor to premature ageing. Therefore, not only can we argue that following a routine capable of neutralising these effects is crucial, but we can also declare that sun protection is the core of every anti-aging routine.

Therefore, include these 10 anti-aging skin care strategies in your regimen to treat visible indications of aging and enhance moisture.

1. Wash With a Cream Cleanser: Regardless of your age, skin type, or skin issues, everyday washing is necessary. If you have noticeably aged skin, look for a nourishing cream cleanser rather than a foamy one as they tend to be harsh on the face and dry it out. As skin ages, it loses moisture, nutrients, and natural oils, resulting in skin that appears and feels dry. A cream cleanser can refill moisture on the surface of the skin without leaving it feeling tight and stripped after usage.

2. Exfoliate Weekly: There are a variety of advantages that come with frequent exfoliation. Those include eliminating dead skin cells, unclogging pores, and whitening the skin, which is why it's such an important element of any anti-aging skin care program.

One to three times a week, replace your cream cleanser with a light exfoliating cleanser. Pay attention to how your skin reacts after using it to establish the frequency that works best for you.

3. Apply a Facial Serum: Once you've washed your skin, you're ready to apply a face serum that may treat any skin troubles you may have.
As you age, cell regeneration slows down, producing a loss in your skin's overall vitality and luminosity. With repeated application over time, this luscious serum helps skin to appear and feel smoother, firmer, better moisturised, and noticeably rejuvenated. For optimal results, pat the serum over a clean face morning and night.

4. Use a Targeted Eye Cream: In case you weren't aware, the sensitive skin around your eyes requires treatment regardless of your age. Choose a mixture that may treat the apparent indications of ageing you notice around your eyes and nourishing vitamin E. Morning and night, use your ring finger to massage the product gently around the eye region until it's well absorbed.

5. Moisturise With Your Skin Type in Mind: Let it be known that all skin types require hydration. Mature skin tends to be dry, which means a rich, moisturising moisturiser may assist enhance the way your skin looks and feels.

6. Try a Facial Oil: Another indicator of aging skin is when natural oil production begins to decline. Daily exposure to damaging UV rays further affects the skin's ability to retain moisture, which may leave it appearing dry and lifeless. That's where face oil comes into play: You may use it after face cream to help seal in moisture for extra skin nutrition.

7. Use SPF Every Single Day: The unpleasant fact is that sunscreen is not going to be vital. But, this particularly rings true when you're putting out an anti-aging skin care program.

8. Remove Makeup Gently: Let's jump to the end of the day: Before you're ready to get some beauty sleep, you'll need to remove your makeup. To prevent the congested pores that napping in makeup may bring, grab a makeup wipe before bed. Gently swipe it all over your skin to remove makeup before washing your face with a cream cleanser.

9. Reach for a Wrinkle Cream at Night: According to the American Academy of Dermatology, sleep offers your body time to recharge and renew itself. Take advantage of that opportunity and apply a wrinkle-fighting night lotion before you retire to bed. These anti-wrinkle face creams assist to minimise indications of ageing, including sagging skin, dryness, wrinkles, and more.

10. Sleep on a Silk Pillowcase: While we're on the topic of beauty sleep, consider how your nighttime routines might also affect your anti-aging regimen. Sleeping on a silk pillowcase may make a major impact on your skin since the silky, slinky texture is kinder than cotton or polyester.

Anti-aging Habits

There are good actions you can do to make your senior years healthier and more pleasurable.

And, they could just add as much as a decade or more to your life.

1. The single greatest thing you can do for your health and life is stop smoking. Smoking has been implicated in a laundry list of illnesses from heart disease to lung problems, all of which might thwart your longevity ambitions.

2. Drink only in moderation. Alcohol permeates every cell, destroying DNA and inflaming your liver. A glass of wine a day for women and maybe two for men, but no more, maybe somewhat advantageous.

3. Consider moderating your overall food consumption. Studies in rodents reveal that a 30% calorie restriction causes longer life (no, it doesn't simply appear longer!). Blackman also cites research in rhesus monkeys demonstrating an increase in years with a decrease in diet. Lowering

extra pounds implies less pressure on your system.

4. Supplement. Most of us suffer from "overconsumption malnutrition" too much of the wrong stuff.

5. Reprogram your perception of old age. Research at Yale recently indicated that people with a good outlook on getting older lived seven years longer than those who griped about it.

6. Get rest and keep off stress. Your body needs downtime to repair cells and relax your heart. And your mind requires dreaming to keep sane.

7. Eat well-balanced meals. In addition to creating obesity, cancer, and other health concerns, consuming too much-processed sugar may also speed up the aging process in your skin, producing dark circles and wrinkles. Save processed meals and

sugary sweets for exceptional occasions and make fruits, vegetables, and healthy grains the major emphasis of your regular diet.

Chapter 9: Exfoliation

Exfoliation is the act of eliminating dead skin cells so that skin appears and feels smoother, softer, and brighter. Our skin naturally exfoliates itself (a process called desquamation), but this process is delayed for certain people and may result in difficulties like flaky skin, rough texture, and congestion.

Skin is a complicated organ with numerous layers. The uppermost layers compose the epidermis, the portion of the skin we can see. The very top layer of the epidermis is termed the stratum corneum. It's made up of 10 to 30 layers of dead skin cells.

These cells are continuously slipping off and being replaced with new ones. A full cycle of cell turnover takes roughly 28 days in younger persons. As you age, the turnover process slows, and it takes around 45 days to complete. Some individuals think that the top layers of skin seem dull or dry, and removing them enhances their skin's appearance. There are certain exfoliating treatments you can apply at home, and a dermatologist or skilled aesthetician may aid with others.

How can exfoliating enhance your skin look?

Exfoliating may enhance the look of your skin in various ways.

According to the American Academy of Dermatology, exfoliation may leave your skin appearing brighter and increase the efficiency of topical skin care products by improving absorption.

Regular exfoliation may also help avoid blocked pores, leading to fewer breakouts.

Long-term exfoliation may improve collagen formation. Collagen is important to beautiful, vibrant skin. The protein also enhances skin suppleness, decreasing the appearance of fine lines and accompanying drooping.

Types of Exfoliation

There are two basic forms of exfoliation, which offer somewhat different advantages for various ailments and different parts of the body.

Physical Exfoliants: Physical exfoliants exfoliate the skin by producing friction produced by seeds or grains inside products, or by equipment (for example brushes, flannels, and pumices). This is great for regions where the skin is thicker or extremely rough, for example on the feet and body.

Chemical exfoliation: Uses substances including acid, retinoid, and enzymes which operate by dissolving the "glue" that attaches dead skin cells to the skin. This is less abrasive and hence is better appropriate to the face skin or delicate regions.

How Properly You Should Exfoliate Your Skin

It depends on which chemical you choose to use, but remember that a little goes a long way. Also, you don't want to exfoliate your skin every day (more on this later).

Using a Physical Exfoliator: If you're using a physical exfoliator, moisten your face first, then apply a nickel-sized quantity of the scrub. Massage it into the skin using circular movements, then rinse with water. Check your product's directions, too – some suggest letting the product on for 30 seconds or a minute before washing.

Using a Chemical Exfoliator: Chemical exfoliators, on the other hand, are often leave-on treatments with no washing necessary unless it's a peel or a mask. Apply one or two pumps to clean and dry skin, and you're set. Again, check the product's directions to be sure you're using it appropriately.

Then apply your moisturiser and other skin-care products on top to take advantage of the greater penetration effect. And don't forget sunscreen. According to one research, AHAs in particular might make skin more susceptible to the sun.

Addressing Common Concerns

Here are the answers to some typical questions concerning exfoliation you should know about.

When Should I Exfoliate?
It all boils down to personal choice and your daily routine.
For example, if you think your skin appears dull in the morning, exfoliating before you start your day may be advantageous. On the other hand, exfoliating at night may help remove any residual makeup or other dirt.

If you use a medicated medication for a skin ailment, you should stretch out the period between that product and exfoliation. Avoid exfoliating if you have wounds or open sores on your skin.

How Often Should I Exfoliate?

Most skin experts advocate restricting exfoliating your face to only once a week since over-exfoliating could cause irritation and damage the skin barrier, leading to increased sensitivity and dryness. The skin on your body is often a little thicker than the skin on your face and, therefore may be exfoliated more regularly. Daily exfoliation in the shower is a fantastic approach to staying on top of dry skin.

What do I do if I have a poor reaction?

If possible, remove the irritating substance from your skin using room-temperature water and mild cleanser.

You should avoid wearing cosmetics or other treatments on the region until the discomfort clears.

Taking an OTC antihistamine may help alleviate redness and itching.

Seek immediate medical treatment if you begin to develop severe signs of allergic reaction. This includes: shortness of breath tongue, throat, or face swelling tightness in your lungs chest discomfort

Can I use a body-specific product on my face and vice versa?

You shouldn't. Scrubs and other exfoliating treatments meant for your body tend to be more harsh than ones made for your face.

Your face tissue is more sensitive than, for instance, the skin on your arms and legs. Using such a substance on your face might result in cuts and other aggravation.

Using a face exfoliator on your body generally won't do any damage, but the solution may not be powerful enough to deliver the results you're hoping for.

Should I consider professional exfoliation?

This depends on your unique skin care requirements and what you're expecting to achieve out of exfoliation. A licensed dermatologist can assist you pick the best approach or product for your skin.
Professional exfoliating procedures include:

Body scrubs: Professional scrubs often include different components than OTC equivalents.

Chemical peels: The fundamental difference between DIY and professional peels is the acid concentration. Professional peels are stronger and may be used with other prescription topicals for optimal results.

Dermaplaning: Your physician will use a scalpel blade to remove dead skin and baby hairs from your face and neck.

Microdermabrasion: Your physician will use fine crystals or a specific rough-tipped instrument to exfoliate the skin and a vacuum to remove dead skin cells.

Chapter 10: Conclusion

I Congratulate you on completing your journey through "Glowing Skin Care"! Throughout this book, we've explored the secrets to achieving radiant, healthy skin and embracing your natural beauty with confidence. As we conclude our journey, let's recap the key points and reflect on the transformative insights you've gained:

Glowing Skin is Achievable for Everyone: From understanding your skin type to mastering the essentials of skincare, you've learned that glowing skin is within reach for individuals of all ages, backgrounds, and skin types. By embracing tailored skincare practices and nourishing your skin from the inside out, you can unlock the radiant complexion you've always dreamed of.

Simplicity is Key: In a world filled with endless skincare products and complex routines, simplicity is your greatest ally. By focusing on the fundamentals of skincare—cleansing, moisturising, protecting, and nourishing—you can streamline your routine and achieve remarkable results with minimal effort. Remember, less is often more when it comes to skincare.

Embrace Your Natural Beauty: Your skin is unique and beautiful, just as you are. Embrace your natural features, celebrate your individuality, and cultivate a sense of confidence and self-love that radiates from within. Remember that true beauty comes from embracing who you are and caring for yourself with kindness and compassion.

Consistency is Key: Building a skincare routine takes time and dedication, but the results are well worth the effort. Stay consistent with your skincare regimen, prioritise self-care, and be patient with yourself as you work towards your skincare goals. Remember that progress takes time, so celebrate every small victory along the way.

As you embark on your skincare journey, remember that glowing skin is not just about appearances—it's about feeling confident, empowered, and comfortable in your own skin. By prioritising simplicity, consistency, and self-care, you can unlock the radiant complexion you've always desired and embrace your natural beauty with grace and confidence.

Thank you for joining us on this journey through Glowing Skin Care. May your skincare routine be simple, your complexion radiant, and your confidence boundless. Here's to glowing skin and a lifetime of self-love and self-care.

Review: I'll Love to Hear From You!

Dear Reader,

Thank you for taking the time to explore "Glowing Skin Care" and embark on your journey to radiant, healthy skin with us. I hope that the insights and tips shared in this book have been valuable to you on your skincare journey.

I am passionate about providing my readers with the best possible experience, and your feedback is incredibly important to me. Whether you found the information in this book helpful, insightful, or inspiring, I'd love to hear from you.

If you enjoyed this book and found it beneficial, I invite you to leave a review for me. Your honest feedback will not only help me improve future editions of the book or other books of similar type but also assist other readers in making informed decisions about their skincare journey.

If you have any questions, comments, or suggestions for how I can better serve you in the future, please don't hesitate to reach out. Your input is invaluable to me, and I am committed to continually striving for excellence in providing you with the best possible healthy living resources.

Thank you once again for your support, and I look forward to hearing from you soon!

Warm regards,
Kristin Hampton